Introduction

Self-care and mindfulness are essential tools for maintaining mental, emotional, and physical well-being.
In this guide, we'll explore practical strategies to help you cultivate a balanced, fulfilling life.

- **Why Self-Care Matters:**
  Self-care isn't selfish; it's necessary for a healthier, happier life. Studies show that regular self-care can lower stress, reduce symptoms of anxiety and depression, and improve overall well-being.

- **Understanding Mindfulness:**
  Mindfulness means being present and fully engaged in the moment.
  It helps reduce stress, enhances emotional regulation, and fosters a deeper connection with oneself.

- **What You'll Learn:**
  This guide will teach you daily self-care routines, mindfulness techniques, and ways to build emotional resilience.
  You'll discover practical tips for managing stress, cultivating positivity, and living a more mindful life.

The Foundations of Self-Care

What is Self-Care?

Self-care involves taking deliberate actions to nurture your physical, emotional, mental, social, and spiritual well-being.

It's about understanding what you need to feel balanced and fulfilled, and making a conscious effort to prioritize those needs.

This can include practices like exercising regularly, setting boundaries, engaging in activities that bring you joy, and connecting with supportive people.

By making self-care a priority, you're investing in your overall health and resilience, allowing you to better navigate life's challenges and maintain a sense of inner peace and stability.

Self-care is not a one-time activity but an ongoing commitment to yourself.

It requires you to regularly check in with your needs and adjust your practices as they evolve over time.

This could mean trying out new hobbies, changing your routines, or learning to say no when necessary. It's also about being kind and patient with yourself, especially during difficult times.

By consistently prioritizing self-care, you build a strong foundation for personal growth, emotional stability, and a more balanced, fulfilling life.

1 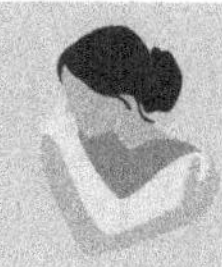

Physical Self-Care:
Exercise, nutrition, sleep, and rest.

2 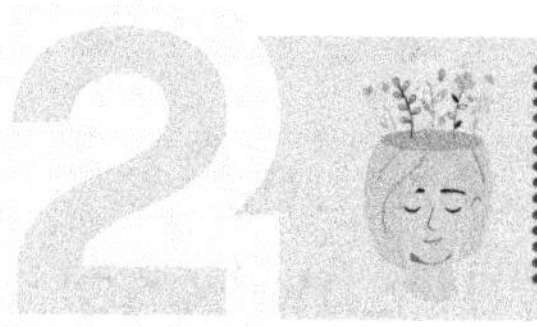

Emotional Self-Care:
Identifying and managing emotions,
seeking therapy, and practicing self-
compassion.

3 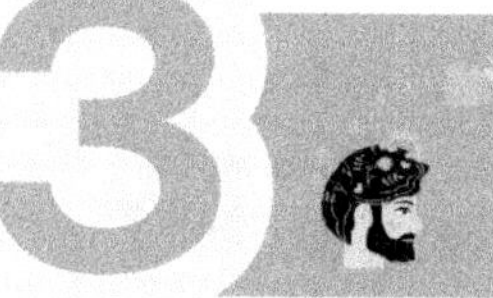

Mental Self-Care:
Engaging in activities that stimulate
the mind, such as reading or puzzles,
and managing stress.

4 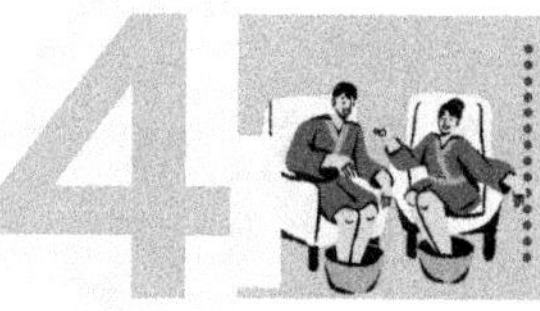

Social Self-Care: Maintaining healthy
relationships and social connections.

5 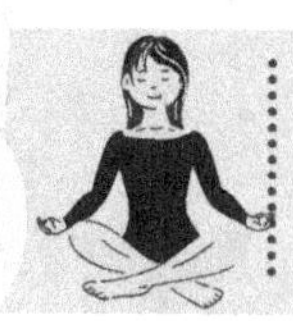

Spiritual Self-Care: Practices that
nurture your spirit, such as meditation,
prayer, or spending time in nature.

Common Myths about Self-Care:

"Self-care is selfish."
Truth: Taking care of yourself enables you to be more present and effective in helping others. It's about maintaining your own well-being so you can support others without burning out.

"Self-care is only about pampering."
Truth: While treating yourself is part of it, self-care also involves discipline and personal growth, such as setting boundaries, prioritizing mental health, and building resilience.

"Self-care is a luxury and requires a lot of time or money."
Truth: Self-care doesn't have to be expensive or time-consuming. It can be as simple as taking a few deep breaths, going for a walk, or saying 'no' to things.

Assessing Your Self-Care Needs:

Use this quick self-care assessment to identify areas where you need to focus:

Do I have healthy boundaries in my relationships?

How do I manage my stress?

Do I get enough sleep and rest?

Tips for Creating a Self-Care Plan:

Set Clear Goals: Focus on specific actions, like exercising three times a week or practicing mindfulness daily.

Develop a Routine: Schedule time for self-care, even if it's just a few minutes each day.

Identify Your Needs: List areas of your life that need attention.

Daily Self-Care Practices for a Balanced Life

Morning Routine for Mindfulness:

1 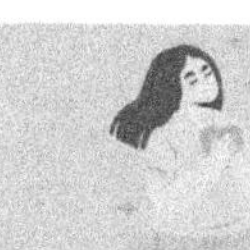 Gratitude Practice: Write down three things you're grateful for each morning to start your day positively.

2 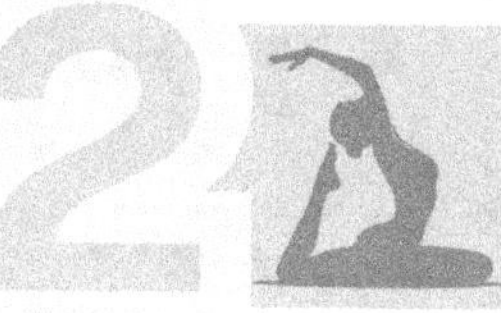 Mindful Movement: Begin with simple yoga or stretching exercises to connect with your body.

3 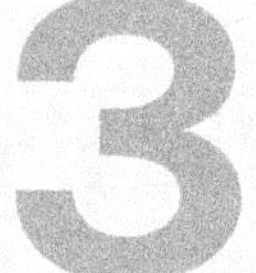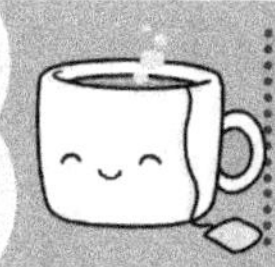 Morning Ritual: Create a calming routine, such as enjoying a cup of tea or coffee mindfully, focusing on its aroma, taste, and warmth.

Midday Mindfulness:

1 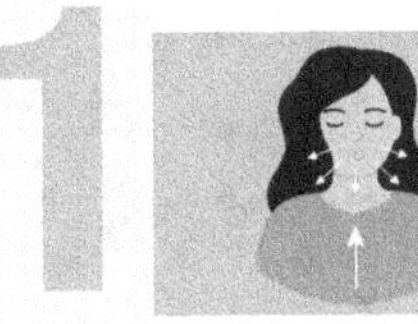 Grounding Techniques: Practice deep breathing or a quick body scan to stay centered during a busy day.

2  Mindful Breaks: Step away from your desk, take a mindful walk, or eat your lunch slowly, savoring each bite.

Morning Routine for Mindfulness:

1 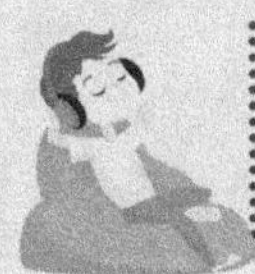 Winding Down: disconnect from screens and relax. Read, listen to calming music, or take a warm bath.

2 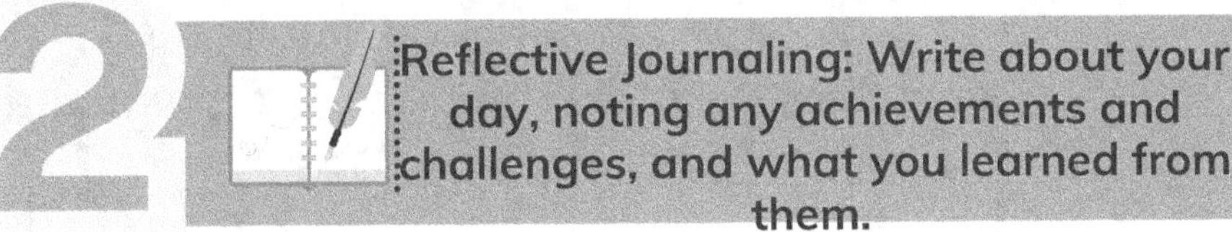 Reflective Journaling: Write about your day, noting any achievements and challenges, and what you learned from them.

3 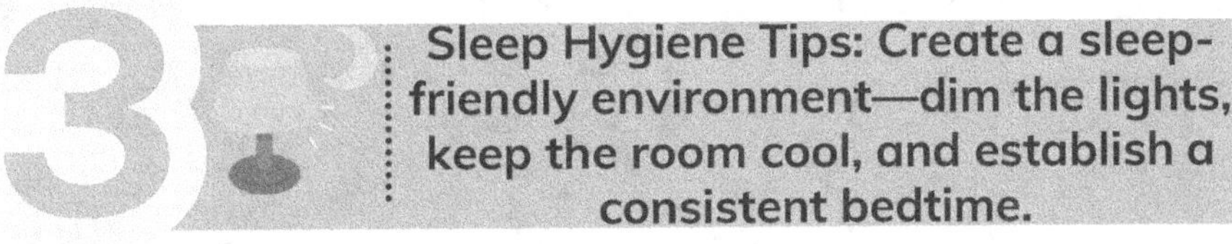 Sleep Hygiene Tips: Create a sleep-friendly environment—dim the lights, keep the room cool, and establish a consistent bedtime.

Mindfulness Techniques for Everyday Life

Mindful Breathing Exercises:

1 **Deep Breathing:**
Inhale deeply through your nose, hold for a few seconds, and exhale slowly through your mouth.

2 **Box Breathing:**
Inhale for 4 seconds, hold for 4, exhale for 4, and pause for 4 before repeating.

3 **Alternate Nostril Breathing:**
Close one nostril and inhale, then switch and exhale through the other nostril.

Body Scan Meditation:

Step-by-Step Guide:

Start from your toes
and slowly move your attention upwards,
noticing any tension or discomfort.

Take deep breaths to release it.

If your mind wanders, gently bring
your focus back to the area you were
scanning, allowing yourself to stay
present and relaxed.

Finish by taking a moment to
appreciate the sense of calm and
connection you've created
throughout your body.

Mindful Eating:

Eat Slowly:
Focus on the taste, texture, and aroma of your food.
Chew slowly and appreciate the meal.

Avoid Distractions:
Put away your phone and eat in a quiet,
calm environment to fully enjoy the experience.

Mindful Movement:

Yoga and Tai Chi:
Engage in slow, deliberate movements while
focusing on your breath and body sensations.

Mindful Walking:
Pay attention to each step, the movement of your
body, and your surroundings as you walk.

Building Emotional Resilience through Self-Care

Understanding Emotional Resilience:

Emotional resilience is the ability to adapt and recover from stress or adversity.

It's about managing your emotions, staying positive, and using setbacks as opportunities for growth.

Being resilient involves emotional awareness, believing in your own abilities, and seeking support from others.

To build resilience, practice self-care, mindfulness, and positive thinking.

Strengthen your problem-solving skills, set boundaries, and maintain a healthy lifestyle.

A sense of purpose and strong social connections also help you stay grounded during tough times.

Resilience leads to better mental health, improved relationships, and a greater sense of control and satisfaction in life.

It's a skill that grows with experience and effort, helping you navigate life's challenges with strength and confidence.

Techniques to Boost Emotional Resilience:

Cognitive Reframing:
Challenge negative thoughts by considering alternative, more positive perspectives.

Self-Compassion Practices:
Treat yourself with the same kindness and understanding you would offer a friend.

Managing Negative Emotions Mindfully:

Acknowledge and Accept:
Notice your emotions without judgment. Allow yourself to feel them without being overwhelmed.

Mindful Journaling:
Write about your feelings, what triggered them, and how you can respond in a healthy way.

Creating a Self-Care Toolkit

What is a Self-Care Toolkit?

A self-care toolkit is a personalized collection of resources and activities designed to support your mental, emotional, and physical well-being.

It can include tangible items like journals, books, or essential oils, as well as digital tools such as mindfulness apps, online courses, and guided meditations.

The key is to fill your toolkit with activities and resources that you find enjoyable and effective for managing stress, boosting mood, and maintaining overall balance in your life.

In addition to individual items, consider incorporating practices that promote mindfulness and self-reflection, such as regular check-ins with yourself to assess your emotional state and needs.

This ongoing evaluation allows you to adapt your toolkit over time, ensuring it remains relevant and supportive as your circumstances change.

By prioritizing self-care and creating a tailored toolkit, you empower yourself to navigate life's challenges more effectively, enhancing your overall resilience and well-being.

Essential Self-Care Tools:

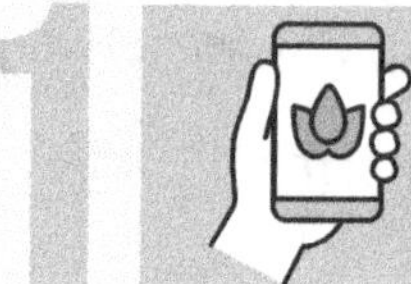

1 Guided Meditations and Mindfulness Apps: Use apps like Calm or Insight Timer for daily mindfulness practices.

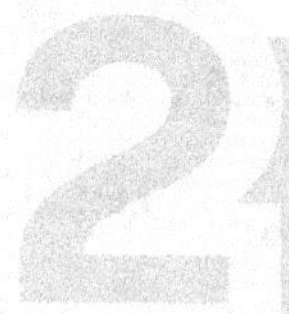
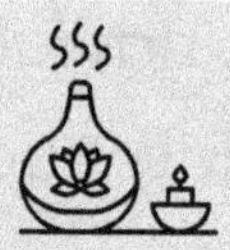

2 Aromatherapy and Calming Music: Use essential oils or soothing playlists to create a relaxing atmosphere.

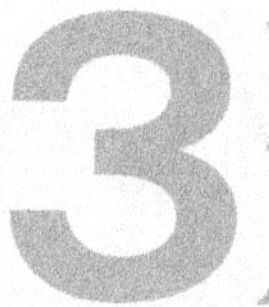

3 Comfort Items: Include things like a cozy blanket, favorite snacks, or inspirational books.

Creating a Safe Space for Self-Care:

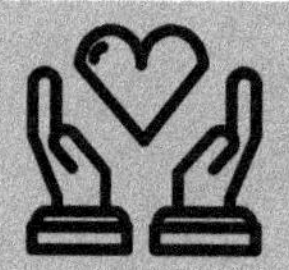

1 Designate a quiet area in your home for relaxation.

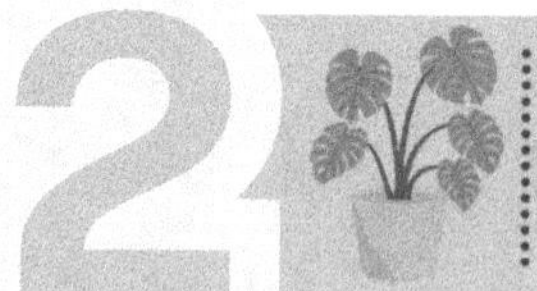

2 Personalize it with items that bring you joy and comfort, like candles, plants, or meaningful decor.

Overcoming Common Self-Care Challenges

Time Management for Self-Care:

Make It Non-Negotiable:
Schedule self-care activities as you would any other important appointment.

Multitask Mindfully:
Combine self-care with daily activities, like practicing deep breathing during your commute.

Dealing with Self-Sabotage:

Recognize Resistance:
Identify when and why you're avoiding self-care. Are you feeling guilty or undeserving?

Start Small:
Break your self-care goals into tiny, manageable steps to build momentum.

Dealing with Self-Sabotage:

Quick Mindfulness Exercises:
Practice breathing techniques or grounding exercises when feeling overwhelmed.

Regular Practice:
Dedicate a few minutes each day to mindfulness to build resilience over time.

Long-Term Self-Care Strategies

Setting and Achieving Self-Care Goals:

SMART Goals:
Set Specific, Measurable, Achievable, Relevant, and Time-bound goals for your self-care practice.

Action Plan:
Break down goals into actionable steps, like setting a specific time each day for meditation.

Sustaining Your Practice:

Reflect and Revise:
Regularly review your self-care plan and adjust as needed to keep it relevant and effective.

Build a Support Network:
Connect with friends, family, or online communities to share your journey and stay motivated.

Conclusion

Reflecting on Your Self-Care Journey:

Taking time to reflect on your self-care journey is an essential part of the process.

It's important to acknowledge the progress you've made, no matter how small, and to celebrate your commitment to prioritizing your well-being.

Consider journaling about the practices that have been most beneficial for you and how they've impacted your mental, emotional, and physical health.

Reflecting in this way helps reinforce positive habits and provides a clearer understanding of what truly supports your overall well-being.

Remember that self-care is not a one-size-fits-all approach, nor is it static.

It's a personal and evolving journey that changes with your life circumstances, needs, and preferences.

What worked for you in the past might not be as effective now, and that's okay.

Stay curious and open to exploring new practices, whether it's trying a different form of exercise, experimenting with creative outlets, or incorporating new mindfulness techniques.

This willingness to adapt and grow is key to maintaining a balanced and fulfilling self-care routine.

By regularly reflecting on and adjusting your self-care practices, you ensure that you're always supporting yourself in the best possible way.

Final Thoughts:

Embracing self-care and mindfulness can truly transform your life, fostering a deeper connection with yourself and enhancing your overall well-being.

It's a journey of self-discovery, where the focus is not on perfection but on progress and growth.

There will be days when self-care feels challenging or when certain practices don't resonate as much —this is all part of the process.

Keep exploring and experimenting to find what genuinely nurtures your mind, body, and spirit.

Be patient with yourself, allowing room for both setbacks and successes.

Remember, self-care is a personal and evolving practice, so enjoy the journey as you create a path to a healthier, happier you.